OCCASIONAL
P A P E R

T0170136

Challenges to Value-Enhancing Innovation in Health Care Delivery

Commonalities and Contrasts with Innovation in Drugs and Devices

Steven Garber, Susan M. Gates,

Margaret E. Blume-Kohout, James R. Burgdorf,

Helen Wu

Sponsored by RAND COMPARE and the Ewing Marion Kauffman Foundation

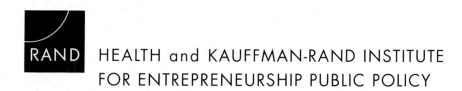

RAND HEALTH and KAUFFMAN-RAND INSTITUTE
FOR ENTREPRENEURSHIP PUBLIC POLICY

The research described in this report was sponsored by RAND Health's Comprehensive Assessment of Reform Efforts (COMPARE) and the Ewing Marion Kauffman Foundation and was conducted in RAND Health and the Kauffman-RAND Institute for Entrepreneurship Public Policy (KRI). KRI is housed within the RAND Institute for Civil Justice (ICJ). Both RAND Health and RAND ICJ are divisions of the RAND Corporation.

Library of Congress Control Number: 2011938451

ISBN: 978-0-8330-5907-9

Published 2011 by the RAND Corporation
1776 Main Street, P.O. Box 2138, Santa Monica, CA 90407-2138
1200 South Hayes Street, Arlington, VA 22202-5050
4570 Fifth Avenue, Suite 600, Pittsburgh, PA 15213-2665
RAND URL: http://www.rand.org/
To order RAND documents or to obtain additional information, contact
Distribution Services: Telephone: (310) 451-7002;
Fax: (310) 451-6915; Email: order@rand.org

Preface

Some innovative health care activities are worth their social costs—or are "value enhancing" or "socially desirable"—and others are not. Health policymakers and researchers seeking to identify and encourage health care innovations (HCIs) that are worth their social costs, and discourage those that are not, face myriad challenges. This paper focuses on innovative activities that increase U.S. capabilities or know-how related to diagnosing and treating medical conditions—that is, "medical technology" broadly defined to include drugs, devices, and methods of delivering health care. The goal of this paper is to provide an early step toward addressing challenges faced by policymakers who seek to promote innovative activities that are worth their social costs and discourage activities that are not.

To accomplish this aim, we develop and apply simple and powerful conceptual perspectives. Our conceptual framework emphasizes effects on population health and national-level costs and adoption as well as invention (that is, creation of new ideas, methods, and so on). We compare and contrast innovation in medical products (pharmaceuticals and medical devices) with delivery to help develop insights about how to promote socially beneficial delivery innovation (DI). The perspectives provided in this paper will assist health policymakers and researchers—our intended audiences—in identifying and designing effective responses to some of the special challenges that confront efforts to foster value-enhancing DI. More specifically, these challenges pertain to implementation, evaluation, policy coordination, and resistance to innovation from powerful stakeholders who believe their interests are threatened. The paper does not, however, recommend particular policy changes.

The development of this manuscript was supported by RAND Health's Comprehensive Assessment of Reform Efforts (COMPARE) and the Ewing Marion Kauffman Foundation. COMPARE receives funding from a consortium of sources, including RAND's corporate endowment, contributions from individual donors, corporations, foundations, and other organizations. RAND Health is a division of the RAND Corporation. A profile of RAND Health, abstracts of its publications, and ordering information can be found at www.rand.org/health. The research was conducted within RAND Health and the Kauffman-RAND Institute for Entrepreneurship Public Policy (KRI), which is housed within the RAND Institute for Civil Justice (ICJ). KRI is dedicated to assessing and improving legal and regulatory policymaking as it relates to small businesses and entrepreneurship in a wide range of settings, including health care and civil justice.

Contents

Tables

Figure

Summary

Limiting the growth of health care costs and improving population health are among the most important and difficult challenges facing U.S. policymakers. The role of innovation in advancing these social goals is controversial, with many seeing innovation as a major source of cost growth and many others viewing innovation as necessary for improving the quality of care and health outcomes. We argue that mitigating the tension between promoting health and controlling costs requires more-nuanced perspectives on innovation and its role in the health care system. We focus on innovation that increases U.S. capabilities or know-how related to diagnosing and treating medical conditions—that is, "medical technology" broadly defined to include drugs, devices, and methods of delivering health care—and we consider innovation in health care financing only to the extent that it may affect invention and use of medical technologies.

Particular innovative activities may or may not be worth their social costs. We refer to activities that are worth their social costs as *value-enhancing* or *socially desirable* and activities that are not worth their social costs as *value-reducing* or *socially undesirable*. Barriers to innovation may be socially desirable or undesirable. Our fundamental premise is that policymakers should attempt to identify innovative activities that are worth their social costs and those that are not and use policy to encourage the former and discourage the latter.

Conceptual Perspectives

To help policymakers consider which innovative activities are and which are not likely to be socially desirable, we propose and apply a simple, but powerful, conceptual framework. The framework confronts two major complications for policymakers, namely, that effects of health care and health care innovation (HCI) are realized over many years and that these effects are uncertain at the time that policymakers choose their actions. To address the former, we define outcomes in terms of trajectories over time and use (mathematically) expected values to represent uncertain outcomes.

More specifically, we define the (social) value of health care as the difference between the time-discounted future trajectories of the expected values of (1) population health, measured for each time period as population-level aggregate quality-adjusted life years, and (2) total social costs of resources devoted to health care. Accordingly, we define the social value of HCI in the aggregate or of particular innovative activities as the expected change in the social value of health care attributable to innovation. In other words, the social value of an innovative activity is the difference between the resulting changes in (mathematically expected and time-discounted) population health and aggregate health care costs.

We apply this framework to consider a variety of policy issues pertaining to innovation in pharmaceuticals, medical devices, and health care delivery—three domains that are typically considered in isolation. Drawing upon and synthesizing wide-ranging literature, we discuss commonalities and contrasts between drugs and devices on the one hand and delivery on the other.

The Importance of Delivery Innovation

We emphasize delivery innovation (DI) for several reasons, including the following. The Institute of Medicine's (IOM's) (2001) *Crossing the Quality Chasm* suggests that DI is lagging behind other kinds of HCI, and that DI may have great potential for increasing quality, reducing costs, or both. Moreover, enhancing social value through commercialization and adoption of DIs has proved to be very challenging—seemingly much more so than for drugs and devices—because of difficulties in effectively implementing promising inventions.

Cross-Cutting Perspectives

Some conceptual perspectives that we develop in this paper pertain broadly to drugs, devices, and delivery, and we begin by discussing them. For example, we propose a system for prioritizing HCIs for policy attention, discuss tensions between promoting social value in the short and long runs, and introduce the "value chasm," which generalizes the IOM's "quality chasm" to include social costs along with the quality of care.

Issues Specific to Drugs and Devices

We also discuss some issues that are largely specific to drugs and devices. For example, we emphasize that the social value of drug and device innovation depends on how much and how the drugs and devices are used, thereby highlighting the potential influence of DI on the social value of drug and device innovation. We also review literature pertaining to social tradeoffs related to patentability.

Varieties of Delivery Innovation

There are a wide variety of DIs, and there appears to be no widely accepted taxonomy. This lack of a taxonomy may impede understanding of the challenges to DI, which may differ across categories of such innovations. In this paper, we take some steps toward developing such a taxonomy. We highlight and discuss several categories of DIs that are not nearly as widely adopted as they may become. These DIs include those intended to improve the quality of care management for patients with chronic diseases, such as the Chronic Care Model and disease management programs; innovations in health information technology; and new settings for delivering care, such as retail health clinics and specialty hospitals.

Market- and Policy-Based Obstacles to Value-Enhancing Innovation

Furthermore, we discuss factors that appear to impede the potential of innovation to enhance the value of health care. Many of these obstacles to value-enhancing HCI fall into seven categories that pertain to drugs and devices as well as delivery. As detailed in Table S.1, these categories fall into two major groups, namely, market imperfections (imperfect information, externalities, and lack of effective competition) and policy choices (payment, regulations, tort liability, and budget pressures). Table S.1 provides selected examples of obstacles falling into the seven categories for drugs and devices (the second column) and delivery (the third column). Additionally, we highlight two obstacles to improving the social value of DI that are largely specific to DI, namely, (1) the need for coordination across distinct public and private policymakers and (2) resistance to innovation from powerful stakeholders who believe their interests are threatened.

The Value Chasm in Theory and in Practice

Increasing the degree to which innovation in health care delivery promotes social value is critical to improving the overall performance of the U.S. health care system. As for the quality chasm, the value chasm pertains to gaps between what is possible in theory and what is achieved in practice. Difficulties in implementing DIs suggest, however, that the value actually realized from DI will often fall short of what is possible in principle. Policymakers who do not consider likely implementation difficulties will be unrealistically optimistic about the expected social value of many DIs.

Challenges for Policymakers in Enhancing Value Through Delivery Innovation

Intentionally and otherwise, federal, state, and private policymakers affect the levels and directions of innovative activities related to health care delivery by promoting or hindering innovative activities of different kinds. In the final chapter of the paper, we use insights from our analysis of selected DIs to consider the market and policy challenges to value-enhancing DI in greater depth.

Policymakers actively seeking to enhance the social value of DI confront several formidable challenges. Perhaps the most daunting challenges are (1) identifying DI activities to be encouraged or discouraged; (2) designing effective, feasible policy responses; and (3) garnering the required support to put such policies into effect.

Improving the social value of DI will require sustained efforts by both policymakers and policy researchers. Researchers can help policymakers identify DI activities that are and those that are not likely to be socially desirable, suggest promising policy actions, and predict how different public policies are likely to affect the mix of innovative activities.

As public policymakers confront such daunting challenges, private actors may also play major roles in shaping the future of DI. The role of private entrepreneurs in promoting DI, which has not been extensively studied, may also be crucial in shaping the future contours of U.S. health care.

Table S.1
Selected Obstacles to Value-Enhancing Health Care Innovation and Selected Examples

Obstacles	Drugs and Devices	Delivery
Market Imperfections		
Imperfect information	Lack of cost-effectiveness information for key subpopulations	Exceptional difficulty of assessing many DIs
	Inadequate incentives to produce or disseminate cost-effectiveness information	Major variation in implementation of many DIs
	Assessments substantially lag technological changes	
Externalities	Imitation undermines incentives to invent	Uncertain property rights for methods of service
		Network effects of health information technologies
Lack of effective competition	Limited price competition among manufacturers	Quality and price competition among providers often ineffective
	Quality competition among providers often ineffective	Little competition on convenience or price transparency
Policy Choices		
Payment	Tension between marginal and average costs	Fee-for-service payments fail to reward cost-effective activities and offer more revenue for bad outcomes
	Payment rates that do not cover costs of cost-effective products and associated services	High-margin activities tend to encourage competition that may not be value enhancing
Regulations	Costs of some Food and Drug Administration regulations may discourage cost-effective development and use	Awareness and compliance with Medicare and Medicaid rules require substantial resources
		Scope of practice laws can impede cost-effective staffing
		Certificate of need regulations can impede value-enhancing facilities-based competition
Tort liability	Product liability distorts mix of drug development	Use of innovative methods can increase medical malpractice exposure
	High transaction costs of disputing	Costs of "defensive medicine" far exceed social benefits
		High transaction costs of disputing
Budget pressures	Short-sighted decisionmaking can preclude cost-effective investments	Short-sighted decisionmaking can preclude cost-effective investments

Acknowledgments

We thank our colleagues Jonathan Grant, Emmett Keeler, Beth McGlynn, and Jeffrey Wasserman for helpful discussions and comments on earlier drafts, and Peter Hussey for his thoughtful and constructive technical review. Any opinions expressed here are those of the authors and do not necessarily reflect the views of RAND, RAND Health, KRI, or their sponsors.

Abbreviations

ARRA   American Recovery and Reinvestment Act

CCM   Chronic Care Model

DI   delivery innovation

DM   disease management

EHR   electronic health record

EMR   electronic medical record

FDA   Food and Drug Administration

FFS   fee for service

GAO   General Accounting Office

HCI   health care innovation

HIT   health information technology

IOM   Institute of Medicine

QALY   quality-adjusted life year

RHC   retail health clinic

VIPF   value improvement possibility frontier

CHAPTER ONE

Introduction

United States health policymakers are often conflicted about innovation.[1] A widespread inclination to support innovative activities that could improve the quality of medical care and the health of U.S. residents is tempered by a similarly widespread view that new technologies tend to increase health care costs (Newhouse, 1992; Bodenheimer, 2005). Effective policymaking related to innovation in health care is hampered by a limited understanding of different types of health care innovation (HCI) and the influences that policies have on them. Here, we strive to ameliorate this problem by distinguishing among several types of HCI and the policy challenges associated with them. We suggest that mitigating the tension between promoting health and controlling costs—a tradeoff most often considered at a macro level—requires a more micro-level perspective. Our fundamental premise is that policymakers should attempt to identify innovations that are and those that are not worth their social costs and use policy to encourage the former and discourage the latter.

In considering innovation in health care, researchers, policy analysts, and policymakers usually focus on only one of the following areas: drugs, devices, delivery, or a subcategory of one of these domains. Notable exceptions include two reports of the Institute of Medicine (IOM)—*Medical Innovation in the Changing Healthcare Marketplace* (Aspden, 2002) and *Crossing the Quality Chasm: A New Health System for the 21st Century* (IOM, 2001)—and *The Innovator's Prescription—A Disruptive Solution for Health Care* (Christensen, Grossman, and Hwang, 2009). Many of the conceptual perspectives presented in our paper apply to drugs, devices, and delivery; others emphasize interdependencies between drug and device innovation on the one hand and delivery innovation (DI) on the other; and others pertain only or primarily to DI generally or to broad categories of DI.

In the next chapter, we present a simple framework for decomposing innovation processes and defining HCI. Chapter Three offers conceptual perspectives pertaining to all domains of HCI (drugs, devices, and delivery). In that chapter, we define the social values of health care and HCI, present a system for prioritizing HCIs for policy attention, and discuss tensions between promoting social value in the short run and the long run. We then introduce the "value chasm," which is a generalization of the IOM's "quality chasm," in Chapter Four. In Chapter Five, we discuss issues particularly relevant to drug and device innovation, drawing on insights from a large and well-developed literature. These issues include value-enhancing utilization of drugs and devices that were already invented, sharpening incentives for product

---

[1] In this paper, we focus on innovation that improves U.S. capabilities or know-how related to diagnosing and treating medical conditions—that is, "medical technology" broadly defined. We consider innovation in health care financing only to the extent that innovative methods of financing are likely to affect the state of medical technology.

developers to focus on opportunities to enhance social value, and impediments to enhancing the social value of drug and device innovation.

The penultimate chapter applies insights from earlier chapters to consider DI, which has important similarities with and differences from drug and device innovation. We discuss a variety of DIs, including those intended to improve the quality of care management for patients with chronic diseases, innovations in health information technology (HIT), retail health clinics (RHCs), and specialty hospitals. We also discuss impediments to enhancing the social value of health care through innovation in delivery processes. The final chapter emphasizes special challenges for policymakers and researchers in promoting value-enhancing DI.

CHAPTER TWO

Stages of Innovation and Defining Health Care Innovation

Innovating involves doing novel things. Innovation researchers often decompose innovation into three stages. To facilitate our discussion, we use the following fairly common, three-stage decomposition. *Invention* refers to the creation or first occurrence of a new medical product or delivery process or method. *Commercialization* refers to making products or processes available for nonexperimental use. *Adoption* refers to the diffusion or spread of products or processes into use by health care providers, payers, or consumers.[1] While invention is often emphasized in analyses of HCI, adoption is also crucial; after all, an invention cannot affect health unless it is used. And, as we argue below, adoption seems to be especially problematic for many kinds of DI.

We further conceptualize HCI as comprising numerous innovative activities within each stage. We are interested in innovative activities taking place anywhere in the world that can affect U.S. health care costs or the health of U.S. residents. Accordingly, we define U.S. HCI as comprising activities (1) to invent (or create) medical products (i.e., drugs and devices) or delivery processes that could be employed in providing health care in the United States or (2) to change usage patterns of health-related products or processes that are not yet widely adopted or widely rejected in the United States.

This definition of HCI is descriptive rather than prescriptive. Specifically, innovative activities may or may not be socially desirable, and so-called barriers to innovation—i.e., factors that tend to discourage some innovative activities—may be socially desirable or socially undesirable depending on the circumstances. In contrast, it is fairly common in policy discussions for innovation to be viewed as socially desirable and, by implication, all "barriers" or impediments to innovation as socially undesirable.

---

[1] Following fairly widespread custom, we view the outputs of basic—as contrasted with applied—science as inputs to HCI rather than innovations per se.

CHAPTER THREE

Cross-Cutting Conceptual Perspectives

Several concepts are helpful in understanding central issues involving innovation in drugs, devices, and delivery processes and for comparing the social advantages and disadvantages of innovative activities across these domains. In this chapter, we present and discuss such cross-cutting perspectives.

Determination of Actual Innovative Activities

U.S. HCI results from numerous decentralized decisions made by individuals in the public and private sectors, including both public and private research and academic institutions. Throughout this paper, we assume that such decisions are made to further the goals of those decision-makers, which may or may not coincide with the goals or objectives of their organizations or those of society. These goals may, for example, be profits, as we would expect for private, commercial enterprises; and higher incomes, professional recognition and advancement, altruism, or some combination in the cases of individuals. In short, we assume that policymakers can influence the innovative activities that are and those that are not undertaken by changing the opportunities or incentives of the relevant decisionmakers. Most important, since many decisionmakers are not intrinsically and primarily motivated to enhance the social value of HCI, there is considerable scope for our decentralized system to lead to activities that are not worth their social costs and to failure to undertake activities that are worth their social costs.[1]

The Social Value of Health Care Innovation

For policymakers to effectively promote social objectives, they must have a clear sense of what those objectives are. While reasonable people disagree about the appropriate goals of health policy, we assume that the goal is to maximize the net social value of HCI activities. Many argue for improving "value" in health care without defining it, and those who define value offer various, often vague, definitions. Some associate value with health benefits, treating costs as a separate issue (e.g., Nord, 1999), and others emphasize value to patients "per dollar spent" (Porter and Teisberg, 2007, p. 1103), without indicating whose dollars are spent or considering that spending, however defined, can be a very unreliable measure of social cost.

---

[1] Further complicating matters for analysts is the fact that a particular HCI is often the result of cooperative or competitive activities of numerous individuals and organizations.

We define the *social value of health care* as the difference between the social value of health improvements due to care (alternatively, the social benefits) and the social cost of providing that care. Analogously, we define the *social value of an innovative activity* related to health care as the difference between the social benefit of resulting improvements in population health and the social costs attributable to that activity.[2] In what follows, we refer to innovative activities that have positive social value (i.e., those that are worth their social costs) as *value-enhancing* or *socially desirable* and activities that have negative social value (i.e., those that are not worth their social costs) as *value-reducing* or *socially undesirable*.

These definitions, which are prescriptive, are deceptively simple in that they address several issues only implicitly. The following eight comments elaborate on this point.

1. We define "value" in net terms to emphasize that obtaining social benefits from innovation often increases social costs.

2. We define the value of innovative activity in incremental terms because our health care system is too complicated for policymakers to realistically hope to achieve a fully optimal (whatever the social objective) allocation of health care resources. As a practical matter, then, the best we can hope is to identify and implement incremental changes for which the social benefits substantially exceed the social costs.

3. As a descriptive matter, the effect of a particular activity (e.g., a public policy) is defined in terms of the difference between the outcomes that would occur if that activity were undertaken (i.e., with the activity) minus the outcomes that would occur otherwise (i.e., without the activity). For convenience in exposition, in this paper we assume that the alternative to the innovative activity under consideration is the status quo, unless stated otherwise.

4. Effects of HCIs are typically realized over several years. We define the health outcome for any individual as that person's health trajectory over future years and say that an activity improves that person's health if it results in a more desirable trajectory. Thus, for example, an HCI can improve a chronically ill person's health trajectory even if that person's health status continues to decline over time as long as that decline is less rapid or severe than it would have been in the absence of the HCI.

5. Evaluation of health effects requires an explicit measure of health status. We assume that this measure is quality-adjusted life years (QALYs), which subsumes both life years and quality of life (Dolan, 2000).

6. Effects of HCIs are uncertain, and we assume that evaluations of social value are based on expected values given the information available at the time of the evaluations.

7. We assume that health and cost outcomes occurring at different times are made commensurate by discounting to present value.

8. We emphasize societal-level cost-effectiveness analysis as the evaluation method.[3] And we assume that the health measure is the expected present value of QALYs. This implies

---

[2]   For simplicity and clarity, this definition presumes that the innovative activity will, or is reasonably expected to, increase population health. This presumption may not be the case for many HCIs. For example, a drug that appeared promising based on information available before it is marketed could wind up having such severe side effects in clinical practice that its development and adoption would reduce population health. If an innovative activity will, or is expected to, result in a reduction in population health, then the (actual or expected) social benefits of the activity are negative, in which case it cannot have a positive social value.

[3]   See, for example, Gold et al., 1996; Garber, 2000.

that policymakers value QALYs received by different people equally regardless of their incomes, wealth, health status, and so on.

In sum, our definitions lead us to focus on two national-level outcomes of major concern for evaluating the social desirability of various HCIs: (1) population health, defined as the expected present value of the future trajectories in U.S. aggregate QALYs, and (2) the expected present value of national-level health care costs.

Both the meaning and policy relevance of "economic efficiency" in health care are controversial; thus, we do not use this term. In reviewing previous insights and studies that are couched in terms of economic efficiency, we reinterpret in terms of our definition of social value. This change in terminology seems inconsequential for our purposes because the basic insights apply to social value defined in various ways, and the relevant empirical analyses and interpretations seem to apply even if QALYs are valued as they are under our definition.

In sum, increasing the social value of HCI involves fostering or inducing socially desirable decisions by innovators. Throughout, we assume that innovators make decisions to promote their own private goals, which may be profits, benevolence, professional recognition, and so on.

Prioritizing Policies According to Anticipated Effects on Health and Cost

Table 3.1 illustrates a system for prioritizing policies affecting HCI for (costly) attention by policymakers, whose time and resources are limited. This system classifies policies in terms of their anticipated effects—relative to the status quo—on the expected present values of health (QALYs) and health care costs at the national level.[4]

In the table, effects in each dimension are divided into three categories, namely (1) substantial increases, (2) substantial decreases, and (3) insubstantial ("minor") effects. We explicitly refer to minor effects to emphasize that many HCIs are likely to have only small (beneficial or detrimental) effects in at least one of the two dimensions, and such effects might best be ignored in policy analyses to allow more detailed consideration or estimation of effects that seem much more substantial. Thus, for example, the cell in the table corresponding to minor effects in both dimensions is dealt with summarily as "not worth analyzing."

Table 3.1
A System for Prioritizing Policies That Affect Health Care Innovation

Anticipated Effect of a Policy on Aggregate Health Care Costs	Anticipated Effect of a Policy on Population Health		
	Increase	Minor, if any	Decrease
Increase	May or may not be worthwhile	Avoid	Avoid
Minor, if any	Worthwhile	Not worth analyzing	Avoid
Decrease	Especially high priority	Worthwhile	May or may not be worthwhile

---

[4] Most often, it seems, policy discussions of HCI highlight potential means of diagnosing or treating relatively serious illnesses for which innovation could provide large benefits to each affected individual. We emphasize that policies that have small health effects on many people can also have large aggregate health effects.

The other eight outcome cells of Table 3.1 are discussed in groups. First, three cells are labeled "avoid"—these cells correspond to situations in which substantial socially undesirable effects are anticipated in one of the dimensions with no substantial and desirable anticipated effect on the other. Second, two cells are labeled "worthwhile"—these correspond to situations in which it is anticipated that there would be a substantial desirable effect in one of the dimensions and at most a minor effect on the other. Third, two other cells are labeled "may or may not be worthwhile" because they correspond to expected social improvement in one dimension but undesirable effects anticipated in the other; judging whether such HCIs are likely to be socially desirable requires further analysis. Finally, one cell is labeled "especially high priority" to emphasize that policies promoting HCIs that are reasonably believed to offer substantial improvement in both dimensions are likely to receive relatively widespread support in policy debates because they offer something substantial to both advocates focused on cost containment and advocates focused on health promotion.

Social Value of Innovation in the Short Run and in the Long Run

We find it helpful to employ the distinction between the short run and the long run commonly used in economics. In particular, we assume that in the short run, U.S. health care technology—the collection of tools or techniques of health care available for use in the United States or for treating U.S. residents outside the United States—is fixed. In the long run, health care technology expands. In sum, invention occurs in the long run, and commercialization and adoption occur in the short run.

Promoting social value in HCI requires attention to both the short run and the long run. For example, consider a would-be health care innovator motivated by financial returns, such as a pharmaceutical or medical device company. Such an organization will usually invest in a particular activity only if it expects to receive a financial payoff that compensates for its (private) costs of innovation, risk, the time value of money, and so on. Invention of many HCIs requires substantial efforts and costs that must be covered eventually by revenues if the innovation is to be profitable. For example, estimates of the private costs of bringing a new drug to market vary, but in general they are in the hundreds of millions of dollars (Adams and Brantner, 2006; DiMasi, Grabowski, and Vernon, 2004; DiMasi, Hansen, and Grabowski, 2003).

Once a product is developed, however, prices in excess of (short-run) marginal social costs tend to restrict its adoption even if additional adoption is socially value enhancing. Thus, pricing to promote optimal utilization of existing inventions may fail to cover some, and perhaps most, of the costs of invention. And if sufficiently low prices are anticipated before the invention or development activities are undertaken, profit-motivated organizations will not, and even altruistically motivated organizations may not, choose to engage in activities required for invention.

CHAPTER FOUR

The "Value Chasm"

Innovation in health care is viewed as both a key driver of U.S. health care costs—at least in the near term—and as the best hope to effectively meet daunting cost and quality challenges. We see promotion of value-enhancing HCI and discouragement of innovation that undermines social value as critical components for meeting these challenges. A key question, then, is how can policymakers identify and support, or at least not hinder, those innovations that are value enhancing while discouraging those innovations that are not.

A fundamental conclusion of *Crossing the Quality Chasm* (IOM, 2001) is that the quality of health care delivered in the United States—and, consequently, population health—falls well short of what is technically possible largely because the delivery system is poorly suited to take maximum advantage of available technologies. We observe that this insight pertains to health care costs as well as to the quality of care. For example, inappropriate utilization raises costs without improving health sufficiently to warrant those costs. We use the term "value chasm" to refer to our generalization of the "quality chasm" to include social costs along with the quality of care.

Some implications of the value chasm can be seen using the value improvement possibility frontier (VIPF) depicted in Figure 4.1. The horizontal and vertical axes of the diagram measure the expected present values of the time trajectories in U.S. aggregates of QALYs and health care costs, respectively. Combinations of these present values that are technically feasible lie above and to the left of the VIPF. For example, suppose that point A in Figure 4.1 represents the expected outcomes of the status quo set of health policies. Then, in principle, it is possible to achieve the same present value of expected aggregate QALYs at lower aggregate costs (downward movement in the diagram), a higher present value of expected QALYs for the same aggregate cost (rightward movement in the diagram), or some combination thereof. No matter what the dollar value of a QALY, all points downward and to the right of point A and above the VIPF are feasible in principle and are socially preferable to point A.[1]

---

[1] *Crossing the Quality Chasm* (IOM, 2001) focuses on possibilities for moving rightward in the diagram.

Figure 4.1
The Value Improvement Possibility Frontier and the Value Chasm

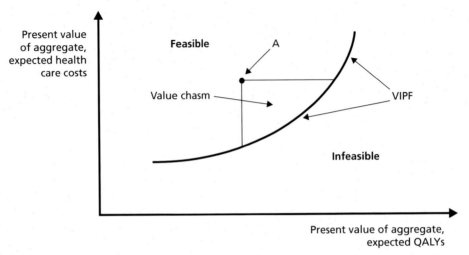

CHAPTER FIVE

Social Value in Drug and Device Innovation

Substantially reducing the value chasm requires additional understanding of numerous factors that influence the social value of innovation. Innovation in drugs and medical devices, on the one hand, and delivery, on the other, also raise several distinct issues. In this chapter, we discuss factors that influence the social value of innovative activities related to medical products. We first discuss issues related to the social value of using existing (or previously invented) drugs and devices, emphasizing (1) that the social value associated with a medical product depends crucially on both how and how much it is used and (2) the social value of medical product innovation may depend substantially, as a result of (1), on features of the delivery system that are determined by past and future DI.

Social Value Depends on How and How Much Products Are Used

Cost-effectiveness analyses of drugs and devices—whether a societal or private perspective is adopted—are usually performed on a per-patient basis and pertain to products that have already been invented. While a per-patient approach is useful for many purposes, it tends to obscure the fact that total social costs of drugs and devices, which include invention or development costs, and their total social benefits depend on how much and how they are used (IOM, 2001, Appendix A; Woolf and Johnson, 2005). The following example elaborates on this point, illustrates that the social value of a treatment (or a product intended to aid diagnosis or prevent disease) is an attribute of technology-patient pairs (not technologies themselves), and emphasizes that improving the social value of drug and device utilization presents major challenges for the delivery system that, in principle, might be met by value-enhancing DI.

Consider treatment of a population of patients with a particular drug or device compared with treating these patients with the best alternative, which for the sake of expositional simplicity is assumed to be the same for all patients. Assume further that for every patient who might be treated, the social cost for the treatment under consideration is $C more than the social cost of the alternative to which it is being compared. Three groups of patients differ according to the change in the expected present value of their members' individual QALY trajectories resulting from the treatment relative to the corresponding changes resulting from the alternative treatment. Finally, assume that additional QALYs have a (gross) social benefit of $v/QALY for all patients.

Table 5.1 specifies for each of the three patient groups the per-patient effect of treatment on the present value of expected QALYs, the net social benefit of treating a patient, and whether use should be increased or decreased within the group to promote social value. Con-

Table 5.1
Net Social Value of Using a Particular Drug or Device to Treat Differently Situated Patients

Patient Group	Cost per Patient Treated	QALY Change per Patient Treated	Net Benefit of Treatment per Patient	To Enhance Net Social Value for This Group
1	C	X > 0	(vX – C) > 0	Increase use
2	C	Y > 0	(vY – C) < 0	Decrease use
3	C	Z < 0	(vZ – C) < 0	Decrease use

sider the three patient groups, which are ordered from highest to lowest expected benefit of the treatment (relative to the alternative treatment), in turn.

For each member of group 1, the increase in QALYs from treatment is X, which by assumption is large enough for the per-patient net social benefits of treatment, namely (vX – C), to be positive. Thus, treating members of group 1 with the drug or device is value enhancing, and expanding use for these patients has an incremental net social benefit of (vX – C) multiplied by the number of additional patients treated.

For each member of group 2, the increase in QALYs from treating a patient is Y, which by assumption is positive but less than the benefit to a patient in group 1. The net social benefit of treatment, namely (vY – C), is negative. Thus, treating patients in group 2 with the drug or device reduces social value—despite the gross health benefits relative to the alternative treatment—and treating fewer patients in this group increases the net social value at a rate of (C – vY) per additional patient treated with the alternative instead. Finally, each member of group 3 receives Z fewer QALYs per patient than under the alternative treatment. Thus, treating patients in group 3 with the drug or device is value reducing, and treating patients in this group with the alternative treatment increases net social value at a rate of (C – vZ) per patient. In sum, depending on the relative sizes of the groups and the degrees to which utilization is beneficial or harmful for the patients included in them, a treatment could be socially undesirable (i.e., have negative social value) even if it is very cost-effective for some patients.

Thus, DIs that would substantially improve how and how much drugs and devices are used could greatly increase the social value of health care. As is widely appreciated, however, this is much easier said than done. For example, it is often uncertain how much a particular patient is likely to benefit from alternative treatments—improved diagnostic procedures could be very helpful in this regard (Christensen, Grossman, and Hwang, 2009, pp. 42–46)—and there are many impediments to reducing somewhat effective utilization whose social costs are too high for utilization to be value enhancing (Havighurst, 1995).

Socially Valuable Invention of Drugs and Devices

There is a fairly rich theoretical and empirical literature on the economics of drug development but little corresponding literature pertaining to medical devices. How aggregate levels of efforts to develop new drugs and devices compare with their optimal levels is far from clear, even for pharmaceuticals.

For example, patents provide temporary monopoly power to drug and device developers and thereby encourage investment in inventive activities. Whether patent protection typically provides inadequate or excessive incentives for drug and device invention is unknown. These incentives may be excessive in some contexts (e.g., for some therapeutic areas) and inadequate in others (Rovira, 2009). In addition, consumers with prescription drug insurance often face marginal prices (co-payment or coinsurance levels) far below the prices received by drug manufacturers, which tends to increase the sales and profitability of drug development. In theory, because patents can confer large implicit prizes to, for example, the first company to develop a breakthrough drug for a prevalent condition, patent "racing" could lead to excessive levels of inventive activity (Loury, 1979) involving, for example, duplication of effort. However, there is little empirical support for this hypothesis in pharmaceutical research and development (Cockburn and Henderson, 1994). Indeed, rather than encouraging overinvestment, in some cases the patent mechanism—specifically, proliferation of basic research patents and strategic patenting by firms—could lead to lower levels of research and development than are socially desirable (Heller and Eisenberg, 1998). Uncertainty about whether reducing or increasing aggregate research and development would increase the social value of HCI does not preclude, however, identification of incremental changes that are likely to be socially value enhancing.

Obstacles to Value-Enhancing Innovative Activity for Drugs and Devices

Numerous forces impede drug and device innovation that is likely to be value enhancing or encourage activities that are likely to reduce the social value of HCI. Removing or lessening these forces could increase the social value of HCI. In this section, we discuss several apparent impediments to enhancing social value through invention (or development) and adoption (or utilization or diffusion) of prescription pharmaceuticals and medical devices. We discuss these impediments within two broader categories, namely, market imperfections and policy choices.

Market Imperfections

Three categories of obstacles pertain to imperfections in the markets for medical products that impede the ability of private markets to serve social objectives.

Imperfect Information. Public and private payers must often decide whether to cover new drugs and medical devices (i.e., provide payment for any of their enrollees) and, if covered, develop and implement rules for approving payment in individual cases. In combination, these decisions largely determine rates of adoption. Often, however, payers confront these decisions without the benefit of much information about effectiveness and safety. Creating and synthesizing such information are the goals of "technology assessment," which is undertaken in the United States by both public and private entities (Garber et al., 2000; Banta, 2003). Lack of adequate information to distinguish confidently among new drugs and devices in cost-effectiveness terms makes it very difficult for payers and providers to separate the wheat from the chaff. Three types of value reduction are likely to result: (1) adoption of drugs and devices that are not cost-effective, (2) failure to adopt drugs and devices that are cost-effective, and (3) (looking to the long run) failing to send credible signals to would-be product developers that the most promising way to make money or to improve health is to focus their efforts on developing technologies that are likely to be cost-effective.

Because cost-effectiveness information, once produced, is hard to keep proprietary, private organizations would be expected to invest less-than-optimal levels of effort in technology assessment. Thus, there is a role for public entities to undertake or finance studies of safety and effectiveness. U.S. government agencies have played these roles historically. The federal role is expected to expand because of $1.1 billion set aside by the American Recovery and Reinvestment Act (ARRA) of 2009—commonly known as the "economic stimulus package"—for comparative-effectiveness research (Avorn, 2009; Steinbrook, 2009; Conway and Clancy, 2009).[1] Public provision of information will tend to promote the social value of HCI to the extent that it produces timely and accurate information that is used by payers and providers. A challenge in this regard is that "rapid change makes knowledge quickly obsolete and places a heavy burden on mechanisms that enable physicians and other health professionals to keep up" (Newhouse, 2002, p. 18).

Externalities. To provide appropriate incentives for value-enhancing medical product invention, inventors would be allowed to capture the incremental social benefits of their efforts. Externalities are a common source of discrepancy between social contribution and private reward. For example, invention of a truly innovative drug or device often lowers the cost of subsequent development of similar drugs or devices, but the earlier inventors are not able to capture the social benefits associated with such cost reductions.

Lack of Effective Competition. There is some price competition among substitute products—for example, different drugs in the same class—especially in the form of discounts from list prices negotiated with relatively large buyers. Social benefits from quality competition among providers and among health plans through more cost-effective coverage and payment policies for drugs and devices seem rather limited, however, because of (1) small numbers of health plans competing for enrollees in many geographic areas and (2) difficulties confronting payers, and especially consumers, in assessing quality differences from available information.

Policy Choices

The remaining four categories of obstacles to value-enhancing HCI pertain to public and private policies.

Payment. Prices received by manufacturers for prescription drugs and implantable medical devices can deviate substantially from prices that would best promote the social value of utilization in the short run or product development in the long run. For example, prices paid (or "reimbursement" rates) to providers by Medicare for injected drugs administered in physician offices or hospital outpatient departments and for many implanted devices tend to be set with an eye toward average—rather than marginal—costs, thus undermining the social value of utilization. Moreover, payment rates to hospitals by public and private payers can be substantially less than what the hospitals pay for implanted devices used in surgeries in their facilities (Garber et al., 2002; Robinson, 2008), thus discouraging use of such devices even when expanded use would be value enhancing.

Moreover, in some instances, payments for devices and associated procedures cannot be made under existing product and procedure codes, or the manufacturer or surgeons are not

---

[1]   Cost-effectiveness research is considerably more controversial and politically sensitive than is comparative-effectiveness research (Weinstein and Skinner, 2010), and the "Federal Coordinating Council, established by the . . . ARRA, is expressly prohibited from setting coverage mandates or reimbursement policies" (RAND Corporation, 2011).

willing to accept payment rates associated with existing codes. Delays in obtaining new codes tend to undermine incentives to develop new products (Garber et al., 2000; Newhouse, 2002).

Regulations. Some features of Food and Drug Administration (FDA) regulations tend to discourage development and wider adoption of drugs and devices. For example, in the long run, FDA regulations reduce incentives to develop new products by increasing direct costs and delaying product introductions; as a result, the number of new products developed and commercialized is likely to be lower than otherwise (Peltzman, 1973; Berndt et al., 2005; Philipson and Sun, 2008). Moreover, in the short run, FDA regulation of manufacturer claims about safety and effectiveness of off-label uses of approved drugs (Stafford, 2008) tends to limit rates of off-label use, which may be value-enhancing in some instances and value-reducing in others. In sum, whether FDA regulations—which undoubtedly prevent many injuries resulting from commercialization and adoption of especially risky drugs and devices—promote or undermine social value overall is unknown and controversial.

Tort Liability. Product liability exposure of medical product manufacturers is sometimes said to "stifle" innovation, but this is clearly an exaggeration since extensive efforts to develop new drugs and devices for the U.S. market continue. Various realities of the U.S. product liability system, however, do suggest that product liability exposure can alter, in ways that are socially value reducing, the relative levels of effort to develop medical products targeting different diseases or conditions (Garber, 1993, pp. 142–167). Moreover, when considering the social value of medical product liability, social costs of disputing and resolving claims (i.e., the so-called "transaction costs" of the liability system) should also be taken into account. As with FDA regulation, however, medical product liability also almost surely prevents many injuries, and whether the overall social effects of medical product liability are on balance value enhancing or value reducing is unknown and controversial.

Budget Pressures. In many instances, it appears that medical product adoption (coverage and utilization) decisions of public and private payers are driven by the desire to control costs. The potential for adoption to be delayed for this reason tends to discourage development activities and may often limit diffusion of value-enhancing products. Diffusion of cochlear implants, which appear to be very cost-effective for children, provides an example (Garber et al., 2002).

CHAPTER SIX

Delivery Innovation and Social Value

This chapter explores issues related to enhancing the net social value of U.S. health care through innovations affecting the delivery of health care. DIs are of major interest for at least four reasons. First, incremental costs and benefits of many DIs depend on the value-enhancing potential of drugs and devices and vice versa. Second, the literature—for example, IOM (2001) and Woolf and Johnson (2005)—suggests that DI is lagging behind other kinds of HCI and that DI may have great potential for increasing quality, reducing costs, or both. Third, enhancing social value through commercialization and adoption of DIs has proved to be very challenging; for example, Berwick (2003, p. 1970) writes: "In health care, invention is hard, but dissemination [i.e., adoption] is even harder." Thus, the degrees to which specific DIs as invented or designed will be value enhancing may depend crucially on the costs of implementing them in practice and the degrees to which implementation approximates the innovations as designed by their inventors. Fourth, as we elaborate in the conclusion, there are several reasons that enabling or fostering value-enhancing DI appears to be considerably more challenging for policymakers than it is for drugs and devices.

There are various diverse types of DIs. Among the most important are innovations that would (1) transform how care is managed for patients with chronic diseases, (2) change how widely and well information technology is used in delivering medical care, and (3) alter the kinds of organizations and settings in which care is provided.[1] We now elaborate on these three categories, which overlap to some extent. In elaborating, we discuss selected DIs that appear to be fairly recent and not as widely adopted as they may well become.

Transforming Care Management for Patients with Chronic Diseases

Delivering health care to patients with chronic diseases accounts for more than 75 percent of total U.S. costs of health care (Bodenheimer, Chen, and Bennett, 2009). It is generally accepted that coordinating care among health care professionals for these patients could substantially improve their health trajectories. It is not surprising, then, that strategies for improv-

---

[1] We know of no comprehensive classification scheme for DIs. Another broad type of DI might include activities that change the roles of various types of medical professionals in delivering care. And if *delivery* is defined sufficiently broadly, another category might comprise various activities to help consumers organize, store, and access their personal health information or to inform consumers about how they might improve their health and health care. This is because such activities will affect delivery through consumer action. Examples include Microsoft's HealthVault, GoogleHealth, WebMD, Keas (Lohr, 2009; McBride, 2010b), and PatientsLikeMe (McBride, 2010a). The diversity of DI is further illustrated by such DIs as different types of telemedicine, medical tourism (Forgione and Smith, 2007), accountable care organizations (Devers and Berenson, 2009; Fisher et al., 2009), and the patient-centered medical home (Rittenhouse and Shortell, 2009).

ing the management of chronic diseases are prominent among efforts to improve health care delivery. We discuss two approaches for doing so, namely, the Chronic Care Model (CCM) and disease management (DM) programs.

The CCM is among the best known and most widely used approaches to reorganizing care in physician offices to improve quality (Leeman and Mark, 2006). The model addresses six areas for action, namely, community resources and policies, health care organization, self-management support, delivery system design, decision support, and clinical information systems (Bodenheimer, Wagner, and Grumbach, 2002). The model does not provide specific rules to be applied in specific circumstances; rather, it provides a framework requiring adaptation to local and other contextual factors. Assessments of individual components of the CCM yield mixed results on cost-effectiveness, however, depending on the disease, intervention, duration of follow-up, and organizational context (Bodenheimer, Wagner, and Grumbach, 2002; Coleman et al., 2009).

DM programs are usually implemented by health plans, often in the hope of reducing costs by improving quality, for example, by reducing the incidence of episodes requiring (costly) emergency department visits or hospital admissions. DM applies clinical guidelines and emphasizes education and engagement of patients as partners in the management of their care (Fireman, Bartlett and Selby, 2004; Leeman and Mark, 2006). One literature review, which relies heavily on other reviews, suggests that DM programs improve processes of care, but it found no "conclusive evidence" for health improvement or cost savings (Mattke, Seid, and Ma, 2007). Moreover, only three of the studies of DM interventions covered by this review involved large-scale interventions of the kinds that are likely to be necessary to have major effects on aggregate costs or population health.

In sum, implementation of the CCM differs considerably across sites at which the model is adopted, as does implementation of any particular DM program. Thus, priorities for policy attention related to management of chronic disease along the lines suggested by Table 3.1 may depend crucially on how a contemplated policy will affect implementation.

Improving the Management and Use of Information

For information to be used to good advantage, medical providers must be able to effectively and economically capture, store, retrieve, and understand it. HIT, including electronic medical and health records (EMRs and EHRs), may offer socially valuable responses to those challenges.[2] Many HITs emphasize the potential to improve various aspects of delivery and thereby improve health, lower costs, or both in several ways, such as reducing errors in prescribing and filling prescriptions, increasing compliance with clinical guidelines, improving diagnostic accuracy (IOM, 2001, p. 164), and reducing waste (Bentley et al., 2008).

While many believe that the benefits of invention and adoption of various HIT-based innovations are likely to greatly exceed their social costs (e.g., IOM, 2001; Newhouse, 2002; Hillestad et al., 2005), such beliefs meet with some credible skepticism (e.g., Himmelstein and Woolhandler, 2005; Walker, 2005). The United States lags many other nations in the adoption of EMRs. In late 2007 to early 2008, only 4 percent of U.S. physicians reported using a "fully

---

[2] The terms EMR and EHR are distinguished by some authors—with EMRs and EHRs used by providers and consumers, respectively—and used interchangeably by many others.

functional" system, with another 13 percent having a "basic system" (DesRoches et al., 2008), and during 2008, only 1.5 percent of U.S. hospitals had a "comprehensive electronic-records system" (Jha et al., 2009). The extent to which limited adoption sacrifices social benefits is far from clear, however. For example, a recent study suggests that use of EMRs in physician practices adopting them has not been nearly as effective in improving coordination of care as many policymakers may believe (O'Malley et al., 2009). In any event, invention, commercialization, and adoption of HIT in the United States are expected to expand substantially because of $19 billion provided for HIT investment by the ARRA of 2009.

New Settings for Delivering Care

Another broad category of DI includes activities related to providing fairly common types of medical care in new settings. This category includes ongoing, long-term trends, such as hospitals providing, on an outpatient basis, services formerly provided only on an inpatient basis and provision in physician offices of services traditionally provided by hospitals. It also includes delivery of fairly focused or specialized sets of services in nontraditional settings, often by new organizations created to provide such care. Historical examples of such nontraditional settings include urgent-care centers and ambulatory surgical centers, both of which have been fairly widely adopted. We discuss presently two other examples that are newer, less widely diffused, and somewhat controversial, namely, RHCs and specialty hospitals.

Weinick and colleagues (2010) provide an overview of RHCs, on which our description in this paragraph is based. RHCs are located within retail stores and are typically staffed by a nurse practitioner and, much less often, a physician or a physician's assistant. RHCs provide alternatives to physician office visits for a small number of minor acute conditions and some preventative services, such as immunizations. It appears, however, that some RHC companies are expanding into management of chronic diseases. RHCs offer more convenience than most physician practices by providing evening and weekend services and not requiring appointments. They also offer price transparency, which is fairly uncommon with many other health care services. The first U.S. RHC opened in 2000, and they now number more than 1,000. Nearly three-quarters of them are owned and operated by the parent company of the retail store that houses the clinic. In 2010, 33 states had at least one RHC. The extent to which RHCs represent a competitive threat to physicians is unknown and controversial. Effects of RHCs on health and health care costs have not been studied extensively, although research has shown that for some common conditions, RHCs deliver equivalent quality care at a lower cost (Mehrotra et al., 2009).

Controversy about cardiac, orthopedic, and surgical specialty hospitals at least partially owned by physicians ("physician-owned specialty hospitals") resulted in an 18-month moratorium imposed in the Medicare Prescription Drug, Improvement and Modernization Act of 2003. The policy issues, controversies, and surrounding politics are described by the General Accounting Office (GAO) (2003), Inglehart (2005), Shactman (2005), and Guterman (2006). Opponents of specialty hospitals, including the American Hospital Association and the Federation of American Hospitals, cite three major concerns, namely, (1) threats to the financial viability of general and community hospitals and their ability to cross-subsidize unprofitable (including uncompensated or charity) care due to specialty hospitals diverting relatively profitable services and patients ("cream skimming" or "cherry picking"), (2) lack of emergency departments in many specialty hospitals, and (3) potential increases in inappropriate utilization resulting from physicians' financial incentives to refer patients to facilities in which they have ownership interests. In 2001, there were roughly 60 cardiac, orthopedic, and surgical (not necessarily physician owned) specialty hospitals in the United States (GAO, 2003, Table 2). According to the Physician Hospitals of America, there were 265 physician-owned hospitals in the United States, including 149 "multispecialty" hospitals (Silva, 2010). Virtually all of the specialty hospitals opened from 1990 to 2003 were located in states without certificate of need regulations (GAO, 2003, p. 15). A recent, major policy development is that section 6001 of the federal Patient Protection and Affordable Care Act of 2010 bars both Medicare participation by physician-owned specialty hospitals not certified for participation by the end of 2009 and expansion of existing certified facilities (Silva, 2010).

Obstacles to Value-Enhancing Delivery Innovation

Many obstacles to value-enhancing DI fall into the same seven categories that we used to classify obstacles to value-enhancing drug and device innovation. And as with the discussion of obstacles for drugs and devices, we classify obstacles to value-enhancing DI according to whether they pertain to market imperfections or policy choices.[3]

Market Imperfections

Three categories of obstacles pertain to imperfections in the markets for health care products and services that impede the ability of private markets to promote the net social value of DI.

Imperfect Information. There is substantial uncertainty about the costs and potential health benefits of many DIs, including the CCM, DM programs, various kinds of HIT, RHCs, and specialty hospitals, making it more difficult to identify value-enhancing activities and particularly cost-effective measures. These uncertainties limit opportunities to advance social objectives through markets. Moreover, as discussed in the conclusion, such uncertainties also make it difficult for public policymakers to identify value-enhancing activities and cost-effective means of encouraging them. DIs such as the CCM are difficult to evaluate in cost-effectiveness terms from observational studies[4] because of substantial variation in implementation, including which of the CCM components are adopted, the intensities of the changes, and fidelity to sustained change (Cretin, Shortell, and Keeler, 2004; Pearson et al., 2005). Similarly, it is challenging to evaluate the health and cost consequences of HIT because of variation in what kinds of HIT systems are adopted, how well they are implemented, and how they are used in delivering care. As for drugs and devices, the state of knowledge about the effectiveness of various DIs is expected to improve because some of the $1.1 billion set aside by the ARRA of 2009 for comparative-effectiveness research is to be used to study delivery processes (Conway and Clancy, 2009).

Externalities. As with drugs and devices, there are several reasons that the full social benefits of DI activities cannot be captured by the responsible innovators, thus undermining incentives for undertaking value-enhancing activities. For example, invention of an improved

---

[3]   It also appears, however, that there are major impediments in the delivery context that do not have important analogs in the context of drugs and devices; we discuss these subsequently.

[4]   It seems that DIs are rarely subjected to randomized controlled trials.

method for managing chronic illnesses is costly, and financial incentives to undertake such efforts can be undermined if others can imitate the innovation without paying the inventor.[5] In contrast, while invention may typically be more costly for drugs and some devices than invention of new methods of delivery, patents generally afford inventors of drugs and devices substantial ability to appropriate much of the social value of their creations.

In the context of HIT, some of the social benefits of adoption are "network effects" (a particular form of positive externalities) whereby "each user's . . . incentive to adopt, increases as more others adopt" (Farrell and Klemperer, 2007, p. 1974). In the presence of network effects, adopters do not capture the full social benefits of their adoption decisions. Lack of widespread agreement on technical standards fostering interoperability or technical compatibility between HIT systems is one of the most commonly cited barriers to wider HIT implementation (Hersh, 2004; Bates, 2005; Jha et al., 2009). Overcoming this barrier could have major benefits in terms of spurring adoption of value-enhancing HITs, but much of the social benefit of such standards may accrue to others than the individuals and organizations responsible for the development of the standards. A major government role in standardization is controversial, however, because of concerns about impeding innovative activity by private entities (Blumenthal, 2006).

Lack of Effective Competition. Enhancing the value of U.S. health care through DI is also impeded by lack of effective competition. The dimensions of competition receiving the most attention are price and quality. Attaining potential social benefits from such competition is limited by (1) difficulties in measuring differences in quality, especially for fairly small provider organizations or for all but the most common health conditions; (2) challenges in informing payers and consumers about quality differences across plans and providers in sufficiently detailed but nonetheless understandable ways; (3) lack of price competition in many markets; (4) insured consumers being responsible for only a part of the full price of services they receive; and (5) payers such as employers and insurers valuing tradeoffs between price and quality differently than is consistent with value-enhancing social tradeoffs. In contrast to the widespread emphasis on price and quality competition, RHCs appear to compete effectively with physician offices on dimensions that do not receive much attention in the literature, namely, convenience and price transparency.

Policy Choices

The next four categories of obstacles to value-enhancing HCI pertain to public and private policies.

Payment. Policies that misalign payment with social benefits tend to undermine value-enhancing DI. Many have noted aspects of fee-for-service (FFS) payment that fail to reward behavior that is cost-effective or that encourage behavior that is not. For example, in the context of innovative approaches to chronic care management, including the CCM, there is often no separate payment for costly activities widely believed to be value enhancing, such as team

---

[5] The fact that non-inventors may benefit greatly from imitating inventors of some DIs may be viewed as a "free-rider" problem. The patentability of particular, novel business or service methods—including methods of delivering health care services—is far from clear. More specifically, the 2010 U.S. Supreme Court decision in *Bilski v. Kappos* established that some business methods are patentable but left considerable uncertainty about the circumstances under which particular methods are patentable (Samuelson and Schultz, 2011; Raysman and Brown, 2011). Moreover, enforcing patents by suing infringers is often costly and risky. Thus, inventors of novel ways for delivering health care services cannot be confident that they can use patents to exclude others from using the methods they create.

meetings, other activities related to care coordination, and emailing with patients (Coleman et al., 2009). Moreover, failures of chronic care can result in demand for additional services that are covered by FFS payment schedules, thus resulting in increased revenues for providers. In the context of HIT, there may be funds available to subsidize the up-front costs of purchasing hardware, software, and networking services as well as training office or hospital staff to use the systems—such as those to be made available through the economic stimulus program— but these subsidies will not cover the costs of ongoing upgrades and support. Moreover, providers that invest resources to adopt HIT may as a result face decreased revenues under FFS arrangements if their HIT use reduces utilization of services for which payments are available. The 2010 restrictions on Medicare certification—and, thus, Medicare payment—for new or newly expanded physician-owned specialty hospitals may or may not impede value enhancement. This depends on whether the additional capacity preempted would be socially cost-effective, which is unknown.

A potentially promising response to the disadvantages of paying for some health care services and not others is to institute bundled payment schemes that involve paying for episodes of care rather than paying for individual services. A bundled-payment approach would encourage providers to adopt cost-effective strategies (Luft, 2009). Bundled payment, however, also provides incentives to reduce levels of value-enhancing care along with value-reducing care; see, for example, Pham and colleagues (2010), who also describe complexities in designing an effective bundled-payment system.

Lastly, misalignment of payment with marginal costs of providing services can create incentives for providers to specialize in, and expand utilization of, services that are more profitable whether or not they are value enhancing. This possibility is a central issue in the debate about specialty hospitals and "cream skimming" or "cherry picking." The extent to which specialty hospitals enhance or undermine the social value of health care is unknown, however.

Regulations. Health care delivery is regulated in numerous ways, and regulations can impede value-enhancing DI. At the federal level, the direct costs of reviewing, understanding and complying with "130,000 pages of [Centers for Medicare & Medicaid Services] rules, regulations and guidelines" are considerable (Aspden, 2002, p. 37), and various parts of these costs may or may not be outweighed by the corresponding social benefits. Moreover, "scope of practice laws" in various states specify the services each type of medical professional (e.g., physicians, registered nurses) may legally perform. These regulations have been criticized for inhibiting flexible, creative, and value-enhancing use of lower-cost nonphysician caregivers such as nurse practitioners (IOM, 2001, pp. 214–218; Jost and Emanuel, 2008; Robinson and Smith, 2008). If the social benefits of such regulations, which are often aimed at protecting patient safety and ensuring quality care, do not exceed their social costs, then they tend to undermine value-enhancing DI. Finally, certificate of need regulations, which apparently prevented the introduction of specialty hospitals in some states, may or may not have been value enhancing in this context, depending on the social cost-effectiveness of such facilities.

Tort Liability. In the context of DI, the key form of tort liability is liability for medical malpractice. One form of value-reducing response to liability exposure is "defensive medicine," a term used to refer to care that is delivered primarily for the legal protection of providers rather than for health benefits to their patients and thus is likely to increase costs with little, if any, accompanying improvement in health. While the existence of defensive medicine seems largely uncontroversial, its aggregate social costs have not been reliably quantified and remain controversial (Danzon, 2000; Mello and Brennan, 2009). Moreover, and perhaps more important, since a legal finding of liability typically requires a deviation from custom or the "standard of care," medical malpractice tends to discourage innovative approaches to delivering care (Danzon, 2000; IOM, 2001, pp. 218–219). Finally, as with product liability, the social costs of the medical malpractice system include the direct or transaction costs of disputing and resolving claims.

Budget Pressures. The potential for failure to make costly investments in implementing value-enhancing DIs, such as innovative approaches to chronic-care management and HIT, is higher when payers and providers are under greater pressure to limit costs in the short run. Moreover, much of the resistance to the spread of physician-owned specialty hospitals—which may or may not be value enhancing—is rooted in financial pressures on incumbent community and general hospitals.[6]

Impediments Largely Specific to Delivery Innovation

Two major impediments to value-enhancing DI that seem not to fit neatly into any of the seven categories also seem relatively unimportant in the context of drugs and devices.

Need to Coordinate. First, effective adoption of many kinds of DIs—such as methods for improving management of chronic diseases and many kinds of HIT—appear to require coordination across several actors and organizations. When effective coordination is achieved, the costs of coordination may be very high, and when adoption is attempted but coordination is not achieved, actual social benefits may fall far short of the levels that are technically possible.

Threats to Powerful Stakeholders. Some forms of DI represent major threats to the private interests of incumbent stakeholders; examples include specialty hospitals and RHCs. Powerful stakeholders can be expected to try, and sometimes succeed, to prevent value-enhancing DIs that they view as threats to their interests.

The Value Chasm in Theory and Practice

The existence of a quality chasm was explained at the beginning of the Executive Summary to IOM (2001, p. 1):

> The American health care delivery system is in need of fundamental change. Many patients, doctors, nurses, and health care leaders are concerned that the care delivered is not, essentially, the care we should receive. . . . Americans should be able to count on receiving care that meets their needs and is based on the best scientific knowledge.

The "chasm," then, appears to pertain to gaps between what is theoretically possible and what is achieved in practice and does not address costs of improving delivery or value enhancement. Among the relevant costs are costs of adoption, and such costs—along with failures of replication or faithful adoption—may imply that many DIs that are theoretically value enhancing will, in practice, be value reducing. Thus, much is yet to be learned about the nature and extent of the "value chasm" in health care delivery.

---

[6]   Budget pressures could also spur cost-saving DIs that are value enhancing, particularly when cost reduction does not lead to revenue decreases.

CHAPTER SEVEN

Conclusion

In this paper, we compare and contrast DI with drug and device innovation to develop insights about whether and why DI is lagging behind drug and device innovation. We argue that it is more instructive for policy purposes to consider these questions not relative to what is technically possible, but rather in terms of the degrees to which value-enhancing opportunities are effectively exploited and value-reducing activities are avoided. It appears that the difficulties, costs, and risks of adoption are more often crucial for delivery than for drugs and devices.

Obtaining substantially more value from U.S. health care is of critical importance for both policymakers and citizens, and the future path of DI is likely to be fundamental to achieving that goal. Intentionally and otherwise, federal and state policymakers affect the levels and directions of innovative activities related to health care delivery by promoting or hindering innovative activities of different kinds. They face many challenges in designing and implementing effective policies. For example, much is unknown about the kinds of innovative activities that are more likely or less likely to enhance value and how particular public policies could improve the mix of such activities. Thus, as a practical matter, it seems that the best we can expect from public policy is to achieve incremental, but substantial, improvements. Our remaining comments are offered in that spirit.

Policies directed at social goals other than enhancing the value of DI—such as increasing access to care, promoting patient safety, or reducing public expenditures—might nonetheless have substantial effects on DI. We hope that policymakers focused on other social goals will also consider the potential effects on DI. They may be able, for example, to reform payment and regulatory policies that have counterproductive effects on DI and avoid new policies or policy changes that would greatly discourage value-enhancing DI or encourage DI that undermines social value.

Our final comments are directed primarily to policymakers actively seeking to enhance the social value of DI. These policymakers confront several formidable challenges as they consider how to influence invention and adoption activities, both of which seem crucial. Perhaps the most daunting challenges facing policymakers are those related to (1) identifying DI activities to be encouraged or discouraged; (2) designing effective, feasible policy responses; and (3) garnering the required support to put such policies into effect. We discuss these challenges in turn.

Identifying activities to be encouraged or discouraged is especially challenging in the context of DI. In contrast to the cases of drugs and many medical devices for which randomized controlled trials are possible, experimental analyses of the costs and benefits of many DIs may be impossible or too costly in relation to the potential financial return to innovators. This difficulty should be mitigated somewhat by comparative effectiveness studies and other research efforts. Evaluation of many DIs may, however, await a somewhat wide adoption that generates sufficient observational data to draw reliable conclusions about costs and health impacts. Even more troubling is the likelihood that some potentially value-enhancing DIs that are handicapped by past and current policies will never be attempted by innovators, thereby precluding establishment of their value through successful use.

Moreover, policymakers and researchers should be wary of discussions and analyses of "DIs" that are defined too broadly for them to be studied rigorously. Examples of overly broad DIs include "electronic medical records," "coordinated care," "retail health clinics," and "physician-owned specialty hospitals." Even a more specific innovation, namely, the CCM, allows important variations in implementation, thus making it difficult, and perhaps effectively impossible, to reliably estimate effects. In contrast, a drug that is evaluated for cost-effectiveness is a specific molecule. Attempts to study imprecisely defined activities are likely to result in conclusions that are overly broad, have unclear implications for action, or both.

Once policymakers decide what activities they should seek to encourage or discourage, designing suitable policy responses involves yet more challenges. Effective policy design is hampered by lack of reliable information about the likely effects of different policy actions on what innovative activities will be undertaken. Our best advice in this regard is fairly obvious: Find and use whatever systematic evidence about such effects is available, seek formal or informal expert input, and, if the stakes are sufficiently high and the policymaker has the authority to do so, enable or support activities that will create additional systematic evidence.

A further complication in policy design is that in many instances the most promising policy responses might require cooperation and coordination among policymakers from different federal and state agencies as well as private organizations. For example, enabling widespread adoption of a socially desirable DI might require changes in the payment policies of federal, state, and private payers along with state-level changes in scope-of-practice or certificate-of-need regulations.

Finally, adoption of promising policies may meet with substantial political opposition. A familiar example is that policy measures aimed at cost reduction may be actively and successfully opposed by individuals and organizations focused on improving health outcomes, and vice versa. Another potential source of resistance to value-enhancing innovations is influential incumbents who believe that their interests are threatened by a proposed policy.

When powerful incumbents fail in protecting their interests, the policy outcome may or may not be socially beneficial. For example, suppose that an innovation that would "disrupt" the businesses of incumbents—such as specialty hospitals or RHCs—were widely adopted despite opposition by incumbent providers (Christensen, Grossman, and Hwang, 2009, pp. 82–86; 115–117). Avoiding unacceptable disruption of health care delivery—e.g., avoiding widespread financial distress of hospitals and consequent reductions in quality or access—might require concurrent changes in several policies. Many disruptive DIs may entail major transition costs, with—and especially without—such policy changes. If so, the social costs of the innovation may exceed its social benefits for many years, thereby tipping the balance from value enhancement in theory to value reduction in practice. This suggests a rather discouraging possibility. In particular, disruptive innovation may in truth be "a necessary component to creating a high-performance health care system that is available to all" (Hwang and Christensen, 2008, p. 1329), while the short-term costs may nonetheless outweigh the long-term benefits (when properly discounted to present values). In some instances, then, policymakers may face a choice between facilitating (or at least not impeding) disruption and making extensive and coordinated efforts to mitigate the transition costs—or impeding disruption and precluding, or greatly delaying, the achievement of a "high-performance health care system."

In sum, when it comes to health care delivery, inventing promising new approaches and facilitating effective adoption and implementation are especially challenging. Improving the social value of DI will require sustained efforts by both policymakers and policy researchers. Researchers can help policymakers identify DI activities that are and are not likely to be socially desirable, suggest promising policy actions, and predict how different public policies are likely to affect the mix of innovative activities. In many instances, success will also require coordinating policy changes among federal, state, and private decisionmakers and garnering the political support required to put value-enhancing public policies into effect.

As public policymakers confront these daunting challenges, private actors will also play major roles in shaping the future of DI. Some participants—such as academic researchers and not-for-profit hospitals and insurers—may be primarily motivated by nonfinancial goals, such as professional advancement and altruism, to invent and adopt DIs. But their ability to engage in innovative activities is limited by their financial wherewithal. Other participants—such as for-profit hospitals, health plans, and disease-management companies—will also participate in invention and adoption to the extent that doing so promotes their organizational goals. The role of private entrepreneurs in promoting DI, which has not been extensively studied, may also be crucial in shaping the future contours of DI.

In the realm of "health care services"—one of 17 categories of areas of innovation used by the National Venture Capital Association, which contains many types of DI, but not HIT—venture capitalists tend to support enterprises with few or no earnings (Robbins, Rudsenske, and Vaughan, 2008), suggesting that they support invention and perhaps in many instances also commercialization and early stages of adoption. Robbins, Rudsenske, and Vaughan (2008, p. 1389) report that private equity firms, which include but are not limited to venture capital firms, were considerably more willing to invest in health care service innovation during the late 2000s than they were before 2000. Nonetheless, gauged in dollar terms, venture capital supports drug and device innovation far more extensively than health care services (Ackerly et al., 2008, p. w70). This suggests that investors see much more profit potential over a period of five years or so in drug and device innovation than in many forms of DI. If so, to what extent is the limited profit potential of such forms of DI due to such factors as difficulties in implementation in individual settings and in applying knowledge gained in one setting in other settings, regulatory and reimbursement policies, or challenges faced by inventors in capturing the social benefits of their creations? To what extent is the profitability of DI attributable to value-reducing public policies? These questions are worth investigating.

References

Ackerly, D. C., A. M. Valverde, L. W. Diener, K. L. Dossary, and K. A. Schulman, "Fueling Innovation in Medical Devices (and Beyond): Venture Capital in Health Care," *Health Affairs*, web exclusive, December 2, 2008, pp. w68–w75.

Adams, C., and V. Brantner, "Estimating the Cost of New Drug Development: Is It Really $802 Million?" *Health Affairs*, Vol. 25, No. 2, 2006, pp. 420–428.

Aspden, Philip, ed., *Medical Innovation in the Changing Healthcare Marketplace—Conference Summary*, Washington, DC: National Academy Press, 2002.

Avorn, Jerry, "Debate About Funding Comparative-Effectiveness Research," *New England Journal of Medicine*, Vol. 360, No. 19, 2009, pp. 1927–1929.

Banta, D., "The Development of Health Technology Assessment," *Health Policy*, Vol. 63, 2003, pp. 121–132.

Bates, D. W., "Physicians and Ambulatory Electronic Health Records," *Health Affairs*, Vol. 24, No. 5, 2005, pp. 1180–1189.

Bentley, T., R. Effros, K. Palar, and E. B. Keeler, "Waste in the U.S. Health Care System: A Conceptual Framework," *Milbank Quarterly*, Vol. 86, No. 4, 2008, pp. 629–659.

Berndt, E. R., A. H. B. Gottschalk, T. J. Philipson, and M. W. Strobeck, "Industry Funding of the FDA: Effects of PDUFA on Approval Times and Withdrawal Rates," *Nature Reviews Drug Discovery*, Vol. 4, No. 7, July 2005, pp. 545–554.

Berwick, D. M., "Disseminating Innovations in Health Care," *Journal of the American Medical Association*, Vol. 289, No. 15, 2003, pp. 1969–1975.

Blumenthal, D., *Health Information Technology: What Is the Federal Government's Role?* Washington, DC: The Commonwealth Fund, 2006.

Bodenheimer, T., "High and Rising Health Care Costs. Part 2: Technologic Innovation," *Annals of Internal Medicine*, Vol. 142, No. 11, June 7, 2005, pp. 932–937.

Bodenheimer, T., E. Chen, and H. D. Bennett, "Confronting the Growing Burden of Chronic Disease: Can the U.S. Health Care Workforce Do the Job?" *Health Affairs*, Vol. 28, No. 1, January/February 2009, pp. 64–74.

Bodenheimer, T., E. H. Wagner, and K. Grumbach, "Improving Primary Care for Patients with Chronic Illness: The Chronic Care Model, Part 2," *Journal of the American Medical Association*, Vol. 288, No. 15, 2002, pp. 1909–1914.

Christensen, C. M., J. H. Grossman, and J. Hwang, *The Innovator's Prescription—A Disruptive Solution for Health Care*, New York: McGraw Hill, 2009.

Cockburn, I. M., and R. Henderson, "Racing to Invest? The Dynamics of Competition in Ethical Drug Discovery," *Journal of Economics and Management Strategy*, Vol. 3, No. 3, 1994, pp. 481–519.

Coleman, K., B. T. Austin, C. Brach, and E. H. Wagner, "Evidence on the Chronic Care Model in the New Millennium," *Health Affairs*, Vol. 28, No. 1, January/February 2009, pp. 75–85.

Conway, P., and C. Clancy, "Comparative-Effectiveness Research–Implications of the Federal Coordinating Council's Report," *New England Journal of Medicine*, Vol. 361, No. 4, 2009, pp. 328–330.

Cretin, S., S. M. Shortell, and E. B. Keeler, "An Evaluation of Collaborative Interventions to Improve Chronic Illness Care: Framework and Study Design," *Evaluation Review*, Vol. 28, No. 1, 2004, pp. 28–51.

Danzon, P., "Liability for Medical Malpractice," in A. J. Culyer and J. Newhouse, eds., *Handbook of Health Economics*, Oxford: Elsevier, 2000, Chapter 26, pp. 1339–1404.

DesRoches, C., E. Campbell, S. Rao, K. Donelan, T. Ferris, A. K. Jha, R. Kaushal, D. Levy, S. Rosenbaum, A. Shields, and D. Blumenthal, "Electronic Health Records in Ambulatory Care—A National Survey of Physicians," *New England Journal of Medicine*, Vol. 359, 2008, pp. 50–60.

Devers, K., and R. Berenson, *Can Accountable Care Organizations Improve the Value of Health Care by Solving the Cost and Quality Quandaries?* Washington, DC: Urban Institute, October 2009.

DiMasi, J., H. G. Grabowski, and J. Vernon, "R&D Costs and Returns by Therapeutic Category," *Drug Information Journal*, Vol. 38, 2004, pp. 211–223.

DiMasi, J., R. W. Hansen, and H. G. Grabowski, "The Price of Innovation: New Estimates of Drug Development Costs," *Journal of Health Economics*, Vol. 22, 2003, pp. 151–185.

Dolan, P., "The Measurement of Health-Related Quality of Life for Use in Resource Allocation Decisions in Health Care," in A. J. Culyer and J. Newhouse, eds., *Handbook of Health Economics*, Oxford: Elsevier, 2000, Chapter 32, pp. 1723–1760.

Farrell, J., and P. Klemperer, "Coordination and Lock-In: Competition with Switching Costs and Network Effects," in M. Armstrong and R. Porter, eds., *Handbook of Industrial Organization*, Vol. 3, Amsterdam: North-Holland, 2007, pp. 1967–2072.

Fireman, B., J. Bartlett, and J. Selby, "Can Disease Management Reduce Health Care Costs by Improving Quality?" *Health Affairs*, Vol. 23, No. 6, November/December 2004, pp. 63–75.

Fisher, E. S., M. B. McClellan, J. Bertko, S. M. Lieberman, J. J. Lee, J. L. Lewis, and J. S. Skinner, "Fostering Accountable Health Care: Moving Forward in Medicare," *Heath Affairs*, 2009, pp. w219–w231.

Forgione, D. A., and P. C. Smith, "Medical Tourism and Its Impact on the U.S. Health Care System," *Journal of Health Care Finance*, Vol. 34, No. 1, Fall 2007, pp. 27–35.

Garber, A. M., "Advances in CE Analysis," in A. J. Culyer and J. Newhouse, eds., *Handbook of Health Economics*, Oxford: Elsevier, 2000.

Garber, S., *Product Liability and the Economics of Pharmaceuticals and Medical Devices*, Santa Monica, CA: RAND Corporation, R-4285-ICJ, 1993. As of August 19, 2011: http://www.rand.org/pubs/reports/R4285.html

Garber, S., M. S. Ridgely, M. Bradley, and K. W. Chin, "Payment Under Public and Private Insurance and Access to Cochlear Implants," *Archives of Otolaryngology, Head and Neck Surgery*, Vol. 128, 2002, pp. 1145–1152.

Garber, S., M. S. Ridgely, R. Taylor, and R. Meili, *Managed Care and the Evaluation and Adoption of Emerging Medical Technologies*, Santa Monica, CA: RAND Corporation, MR-1195-HIMA, 2000. As of August 19, 2011: http://www.rand.org/pubs/monograph_reports/MR1195.html

General Accounting Office (GAO), *Specialty Hospitals—Geographic Location, Services Provided, and Financial Performance*, GAO-04-167, October 2003.

Gold, M. R., J. E. Siegel, L. B. Russell, and M. C. Weinstein, eds., *Cost-Effectiveness in Health and Medicine*, New York: Oxford University Press, 1996.

Guterman, Stuart, "Specialty Hospitals: A Problem or a Symptom?" *Health Affairs*, Vol. 25, No. 1, January/February 2006, pp. 95–105.

Havighurst, C. C., *Health Care Choices: Private Contracts as Instruments for Health Reform*, Washington, DC: AEI Press, 1995.

Heller, M. A., and R. S. Eisenberg, "Can Patents Deter Innovation? The Anticommons in Biomedical Research," *Science*, Vol. 280, No. 5364, May 1, 1998, pp. 698–701.

Hersh, W., "Health Care Information Technology: Progress and Barriers," *Journal of the American Medical Association*, Vol. 292, No. 18, 2004, pp. 2273–2274.

Hillestad, R., J. Bigelow, A. Bower, F. Girosi, R. Meili, R. Scoville, and R. Taylor, "Can Electronic Medical Record Systems Transform Health Care? Potential Health Benefits, Savings, and Costs," *Health Affairs*, Vol. 24, No. 5, 2005, pp. 1103–1117.

Himmelstein, D., and S. Woolhandler, "Hope and Hype: Predicting the Impact of Electronic Medical Records," *Health Affairs*, Vol. 24, No. 5, 2005, pp. 1121–1123.

Hwang, J., and C. M. Christensen, "Disruptive Innovation in Health Care Delivery: A Framework for Business-Model Innovation," *Health Affairs*, Vol. 27, No. 5, September/October 2008, pp. 1329–1335.

Inglehart, J. K., "The Emergence of Physician-Owned Specialty Hospitals," *New England Journal of Medicine*, Vol. 321, No. 1, January 6, 2005, pp. 78–84.

Institute of Medicine (IOM), *Crossing the Quality Chasm: A New Health System for the 21st Century*, Washington, DC: National Academy Press, 2001.

Jha, A. K., C. DesRoches, E. Campbell, K. Donelan, S. Rao, T. Ferris, A. Sheilds, S. Rosenbaum, and D. Blumenthal, "Use of Electronic Health Records in U.S. Hospitals," *New England Journal of Medicine*, Vol. 360, No. 16, 2009, pp. 1628–1638.

Jost, T. S., and E. J. Emanuel, "Legal Reforms Necessary to Promote Delivery System Innovation," *Journal of the American Medical Association*, Vol. 299, No. 21, 2008, pp. 2561–2563.

Leeman, J., and B. Mark, "The Chronic Care Model Versus Disease Management Programs: A Transaction Cost Analysis Approach," *Health Care Management Review*, Vol. 31, No. 1, January–March 2006, pp. 18–25.

Lohr, S., "A Web Site Devoted to Your Health," *New York Times*, October 6, 2009, Sec. B, p. 1.

Loury, G. C., "Market Structure and Innovation," *Quarterly Journal of Economics*, Vol. 93, No. 3, 1979, pp. 395–410.

Luft, H. S., "Economic Incentives to Promote Innovation in Healthcare Delivery," *Clinical Orthopaedics and Related Research*, online exclusive, June 19, 2009.

Mattke, S., M. Seid, and S. Ma, "Evidence for the Effect of Disease Management: Is $1 Billion a Year a Good Investment?" *American Journal of Managed Care*, Vol. 13, No. 12, December 2007, pp. 670–696.

McBride, R., "PatientsLikeMe Growing as Pharma Customers Boost Focus on Patients," Xconomy.com, February 10, 2010a. As of August 18, 2010:
http://www.xconomy.com/boston/2010/02/10/patientslikeme-growing-as-pharma-customers-boost-focus-on-patients/

———, "Keas, Founded by Former Google and Bit9 Execs, Tries to Make Online Care Plans Pay," Xconomy.com, June 30, 2010b. As of August 18, 2010:
http://www.xconomy.com/san-francisco/2010/06/30/keas-founded-by-former-google-and-bit9-execs-tries-to-make-online-care-plans-pay/

Mehrotra, A., H. Liu, J. L. Adams, M. C. Wang, J. R. Lave, N. M. Thygeson, L. I. Solberg, and E. A. McGlynn, "Comparing Costs and Quality of Care at Retail Clinics with That of Other Medical Settings for 3 Common Illnesses," *Annals of Internal Medicine*, Vol. 151, No. 5, September 2009, pp. 321–328.

Mello, M,. and T. Brennan, "The Role of Medical Liability Reform in Federal Health Care Reform," *New England Journal of Medicine*, Vol. 361, 2009, pp. 1–3.

Nord, E., *Cost-Value Analysis in Health Care*, Cambridge: Cambridge University Press, 1999.

Newhouse, J. P., "Medical Care Costs: How Much Welfare Loss?" *Journal of Economic Perspectives*, Vol. 6, No. 3, 1992, pp. 3–21.

———, "Why Is There a Quality Chasm?" *Health Affairs*, Vol. 21, No. 4, 2002, pp. 13–25.

O'Malley, A. S., J. M. Grossman, G. R. Cohen, N. M. Kemper, and H. H. Pham, "Are Electronic Medical Records Helpful for Care Coordination? Experiences of Physician Practices," *Journal of General Internal Medicine*, online exclusive, December 22, 2009.

Pearson, M. L., S. Wu, J. Schaefer, A. E. Bonomi, S. M. Shortell, P. J. Mendel, J. A. Marsteller, T. A. Louis, M. Rosen, and E. B. Keeler, "Assessing the Implementation of the Chronic Care Model in Quality Improvement Collaboratives," *Health Services Research*, Vol. 40, No. 4, 2005, pp. 978–996.

Peltzman, S., "An Evaluation of Consumer Protection Legislation: The 1962 Drug Amendments," *Journal of Political Economy*, Vol. 81, No. 5, 1973, pp. 1049–1091.

Pham, H. H., P. B. Ginsburg, T. K. Lake, and M. M. Maxwell, *Episode-Based Payments: Charting a Course for Health Care Payment Reform*, Washington, DC: National Institute for Health Care Reform, January 2010.

Philipson, T. J., and E. Sun, "Is the Food and Drug Administration Safe and Effective?" *Journal of Economic Perspectives*, Vol. 22, No. 1, Winter 2008, pp. 85–102.

Porter, M. E., and E. O. Teisberg, "How Physicians Can Change the Future of Health Care," *Journal of the American Medical Association*, Vol. 297, No. 10, 2007, pp. 1103–1111.

RAND Corporation, "Analysis of Comparative Effectiveness," COMPARE (Comprehensive Assessment of Reform Efforts) web site, last modified March 30, 2011. As of August 30, 2011:
http://www.rand.org/pubs/technical_reports/TR562z14/analysis-of-comparative-effectiveness.html

Raysman, R., and P. Brown, "Process Patents in the Wake of 'Bilski,'" *New York Law Journal*, January 12, 2011.

Rittenhouse, D. R., and S. M. Shortell, "The Patient-Centered Medical Home—Will It Stand the Test of Health Reform?" *Journal of the American Medical Association*, Vol. 301, No. 19, May 20, 2009, pp. 2038–2040.

Robbins, C. J., T. Rudsenske, and J. S. Vaughan, "Private Equity Investment in Health Care Services," *Health Affairs*, Vol. 27, No. 5, September/October 2008, pp. 1389–1398.

Robinson, J. C., "Value-Based Purchasing for Medical Devices," *Health Affairs*, Vol. 27, No. 6, 2008, pp. 1523–1531.

Robinson, J. C., and M. D. Smith, "Cost-Reducing Innovation in Health Care," *Health Affairs*, Vol. 27, No. 5, 2008, pp. 1353–1356.

Rovira, J., "Intellectual Property Rights and Pharmaceuticals Development," in J. Costa-Font, C. Courbage, and A. McGuire, eds., *The Economics of New Health Technologies: Incentives, Organization, and Financing*, New York: Oxford University Press, 2009, pp. 219–240.

Samuelson, P., and J. Schultz, "'Clues' for Determining Whether Business and Service Innovations Are Unpatentable Abstract Ideas," *Lewis & Clark Law Review*, Vol. 15, No. 1, Spring 2011, pp. 109–131.

Shactman, D., "Specialty Hospitals, Ambulatory Surgery Centers, and General Hospitals: Charting a Wise Public Policy Course," *Health Affairs*, Vol. 24, No. 3, May/June 2005, pp. 868–873.

Silva, C., "Physician-Owned Hospitals: Endangered Species?" *American Medical News*, June 28, 2010. As of July 30, 2010:
http://www.ama-assn.org/amednews/2010/06/28/gvsa0628.htm

Stafford, R. S., "Regulating Off-Label Drug Use: Rethinking the Role of the FDA," *New England Journal of Medicine*, Vol. 358, No. 14, 2008, pp. 1427–1429.

Steinbrook, R., "Health Care and the American Recovery and Reinvestment Act," *New England Journal of Medicine*, Vol. 360, No. 11, 2009, pp. 1057–1060.

Walker, J., "Electronic Medical Records and Health Care Transformation," *Health Affairs*, Vol. 24, No. 5, 2005, pp. 1118–1120.

Weinick, R. M., C. E. Pollack, M. P. Fisher, E. M. Gillen, and A. Mehrotra, *Policy Implications of the Use of Retail Clinics*, Santa Monica, CA: RAND Corporation, TR-810-DHHS, 2010. As of August 21, 2011:
http://www.rand.org/pubs/technical_reports/TR810.html

Weinstein, M. C., and J. A. Skinner, "Comparative Effectiveness and Health Care Spending—Implications for Reform," *New England Journal of Medicine*, Vol. 362, No. 5, February 4, 2010, pp. 460–465.

Woolf, S. H., and R. E. Johnson, "The Break-Even Point: When Medical Advances Are Less Important Than Improving the Fidelity with Which They Are Delivered," *Annals of Family Medicine*, Vol. 3, No. 6, 2005, pp. 545–552.